Fit Mom, Healthy Baby

The Prenatal Fitness Guide

Rossana Lewis

TABLE OF CONTENT

Chapter 1: Understanding Prenatal Fitness

1.1 Importance of Exercise During Pregnancy

1.2 Benefits for Mother and Baby

1.3 Safety Precautions and Guidelines

Chapter 2: Getting Started Safely

2.1 Pre-Pregnancy Fitness Assessment

2.2 Consultation with Healthcare Provider

2.3 Setting Realistic Goals

Chapter 3: Exercise Routines for Each Trimester

3.1 First Trimester: Adjustments and Early Exercises

3.2 Second Trimester: Adapting to Changes

3.3 Third Trimester: Preparing for Labor and Delivery

Chapter 4: Cardiovascular Workouts for Pregnancy

4.1 Aerobic Exercises for Stamina and Circulation

4.2 Low-Impact Cardio Options

4.3 Guidelines for Safe Cardiovascular Workouts

Chapter 5: Strength Training and Flexibility Exercises

5.1 Safe Resistance Training During Pregnancy

5.2 Core Strengthening and Pelvic Floor Exercises

5.3 Stretching and Flexibility Workouts

Chapter 6: Yoga and Mindfulness for Expecting Moms

6.1 Benefits of Prenatal Yoga

6.2 Relaxation Techniques and Breathing Exercises

6.3 Mindfulness Practices for Stress Reduction

Chapter 7: Nutrition and Diet for a Healthy Pregnancy

7.1 Importance of Proper Nutrition During Pregnancy

7.2 Balanced Diet Essentials for Expectant Mothers

7.3 Meal Planning and Nutritional Tips

Chapter 8: Managing Common Pregnancy Discomforts

8.1 Dealing with Back Pain and Postural Changes

8.2 Exercises to Relieve Discomforts

8.3 Tips for Better Sleep and Relaxation

Chapter 9: Partner Involvement and Support

9.1 Engaging Partners in Prenatal Fitness

9.2 Emotional Support and Encouragement

9.3 Bonding Activities for Couples

Chapter 10: Postpartum Fitness and Recovery

10.1 Transitioning to Postpartum Exercise

10.2 Recovery Exercises and Timelines

10.3 Adjusting to New Fitness Routines

Chapter 1: Understanding Prenatal Fitness

1.1 Importance of Exercise During Pregnancy

For all of your adult life, you've probably been aware that exercising whether that means a yoga class, bike ride or run can help prevent diseases like type 2 diabetes and benefit your overall health. During pregnancy, there are even more reasons to keep moving or get moving, even if you haven't had an exercise routine in the past. Of course, exercising throughout pregnancy doesn't guarantee a quick recovery or a pain-free back. But health care providers generally recommend that doing what exercise you can while pregnant is a great way to have a healthier and more comfortable pregnancy. (Be sure to get the go-ahead from your practitioner before starting any exercise program during pregnancy. Some conditions can contraindicate it)

Exercising during pregnancy has been found to: Improve Your Stamina and Heart Health: As you may have already guessed, working out can improve your overall fitness. By strengthening your heart and blood vessels through workouts, you're prepping your body to tackle another physical challenge yet to come: labor and delivery.

Reduce the Risk of Pregnancy Complications: Exercising while you're expecting may lower the odds of developing certain conditions like gestational diabetes. And if you do develop gestational diabetes, staying active can help keep your insulin levels in check.

Boost Your Mood: Women are more susceptible to depression during pregnancy, with an estimated 1 in 2 of all women reporting increased depression or anxiety while expecting. But research found that exercise during pregnancy releases endorphins that help improve mood while diminishing stress and anxiety.

Lower Blood Pressure: Blood pressure occasionally does go up during pregnancy, but a significant jump can be a warning sign of preeclampsia. Staying active in one study, simply walking regularly has been found to keep blood pressure from rising.

Ease Back and Pelvic Pain: It's no secret that your growing baby bump puts extra pressure on your lower half, resulting in lower back pain and an achy pelvis. Strengthening your abs, however, may result in less lower-back and pelvic pain during late pregnancy.

Just take care when you hit the gym, and avoid any moves that may worsen backaches (or create new ones).

Fight Fatigue: Low-level tiredness plagues many women during the first trimester, then again late in the third trimester. While it seems paradoxical, sometimes getting too much rest can actually make you feel more pooped. So while you should never push yourself to exhaustion, a little nudge — say, an easy walk or a prenatal yoga class can make a big difference in your energy level.

Improve Sleep: While many pregnant women report having a harder time falling asleep, those who exercise consistently (as long as it's not near bedtime, which can prove energizing) say the quality of their sleep is better and that they wake up feeling more rested.

Relieve Constipation: An active body encourages active bowels. Some women swear by a brisk 30-minute walk to keep them regular, while others say even a 10-minute stroll helps get things going.

Lower the Odds of Delivery Complications: Women who exercised three times a week were less likely to have macrosomic babies (i.e., bigger babies), another study found. Having a heavier baby, in turn, can lead to complications for both mother and baby during delivery.

Speed Post-delivery Recovery: The more you increase your pregnancy fitness, the faster you'll recover physically after childbirth, the more fit you'll be after delivery. In a study, women who exercised recovered faster after labor (even after controlling for the type of delivery), resuming household chores more quickly than those who didn't exercise.

1.2 Benefits for Mother and Baby

Benefits for Mom

Regular exercise throughout pregnancy can help mom adjust to changes in her body due to added weight and changes in hormones, including relief from muscle strain, improve posture and decrease back pain, as well as help battle fatigue commonly experienced in pregnancy. Additionally, researchers continue to look at the role of exercise to reduce the risk of gestational diabetes. They have found mothers who were active before becoming pregnant had lower rates of gestational diabetes later in their pregnancy. Exercise can also help regulate mood swings and prepare mom for labor and delivery.

Benefits for Baby

It makes sense that if mom is healthier during pregnancy due to regular exercise, then the baby will be healthier also. First, mothers who follow a moderate to high intensity exercise regime weekly, tend to better control gestational weight gain. This is good for babies because research has found a link between the mother's weight gain during pregnancy and the baby's increased risk of becoming obese in childhood or later in life. Second, by decreasing the risk of developing gestational diabetes by exercising during pregnancy, mom reduces the risk of labor and delivery complications due to having a larger baby. Finally, researchers also say a mother who is physically active during pregnancy helps give her baby a boost intellectually.

1.3 Safety Precautions and Guidelines

Do not exhaust yourself. You may need to slow down as your pregnancy progresses or if your maternity team advises you to. If in doubt, consult your maternity team. As a general rule, you should be able to hold a conversation as you exercise when pregnant. If you become breathless as you talk, then you're probably exercising too strenuously. If you were not active before you got pregnant, do not suddenly take up strenuous exercise. If you start an aerobic exercise programme (such as running, swimming, cycling or aerobics classes), tell the instructor that you're pregnant. Remember that exercise does not have to be strenuous to be beneficial.

Exercise tips when you're pregnant:
- always warm up before exercising, and cool down afterwards
- try to keep active on a daily basis – 30 minutes of walking each day can be enough, but if you cannot manage that, any amount is better than nothing
- avoid any strenuous exercise in hot weather
- drink plenty of water and other fluids
- if you go to exercise classes, make sure your teacher is properly qualified and knows that you're pregnant, as well as how many weeks pregnant you are

- you might like to try swimming because the water will support your increased weight. Some local swimming pools provide aqua-natal classes with qualified instructors.

- exercises that have a risk of falling, such as horse riding, downhill skiing, ice hockey, gymnastics and cycling, should only be done with caution. Falls carry a risk of damage to your baby

Exercises to Avoid During Pregnancy

- do not lie flat on your back for long periods, particularly after 16 weeks, because the weight of your bump presses on the main blood vessel bringing blood back to your heart and this can make you feel faint

- do not take part in contact sports where there's a risk of being hit, such as kickboxing, judo or squash

- do not go scuba diving, because the baby has no protection against decompression sickness and gas embolism (gas bubbles in the bloodstream)

- do not exercise at heights over 2,500m above sea level – this is because you and your baby are at risk of altitude sickness

Chapter 2: Getting Started Safely

2.1 Pre-Pregnancy Fitness Assessment

A pre-pregnancy fitness assessment should encompass various health checks, lifestyle evaluations and consultations with healthcare providers to ensure that your body is ready for the physical demands of pregnancy and exercise.

Let's have a look at these assessments:

Medical Check-up and Health Evaluation:

- Visit your healthcare provider for a thorough physical examination to assess your overall health status.
- Discuss any pre-existing medical conditions and their potential impact on pregnancy and exercise.

- Review medications you're currently taking and assess their compatibility with pregnancy.

- Undergo relevant medical tests and screenings recommended by your healthcare provider.

Lifestyle Assessment:

- Evaluate your daily habits, including diet, exercise, sleep patterns, stress levels, and any harmful habits like smoking or excessive alcohol consumption.

- Consider making necessary lifestyle changes to improve overall health before conception.

Nutrition and Pre-Pregnancy Diet:

- Consult a nutritionist or dietitian to ensure you're following a balanced diet that includes essential nutrients required for a healthy pregnancy.
- Consider taking prenatal vitamins containing folic acid and other necessary supplements as advised by your healthcare provider.

Emotional and Mental Well-being:

- Assess stress levels and explore stress management techniques such as meditation, yoga, or mindfulness practices.
- Seek support or counseling if needed to address emotional health concerns.

Family Planning and Fertility Health:

- If planning pregnancy, consider discussing fertility health with your healthcare provider.
- Understand fertility windows and factors affecting conception.

Exercise Readiness and Guidelines:

- Discuss exercise plans with your healthcare provider to ensure they are safe and appropriate for pre-pregnancy fitness.
- Obtain guidance on suitable exercises and modifications necessary for your specific health condition.

The aim of this pre-pregnancy assessment is to ensure that your body is in optimal health before engaging in any exercise regimen during pregnancy.

2.2 Consultation with Healthcare Provider

Before starting this amazing journey to parenthood, it's super smart to have a chat with your healthcare provider. Think of it as a check-up to make sure you're all set and ready for a healthy pregnancy.

During the visit, your healthcare provider will:

- chat with you about your health history, any medical conditions, and the meds you take.
- check if there's anything that might cause issues during pregnancy.
- give you tips on eating healthy foods and taking vitamins to keep you and the little one in top shape.

- talk about habits like smoking, drinking, and stress, and ways to manage them for a smoother pregnancy.
- suggest exercises that are safe for you before and during pregnancy.
- if you're trying to conceive, they might share advice on the best times to try.

What happens during the visit?
- You'll have an open chat about your health, lifestyle, and any concerns you have about starting a family.
- Your healthcare provider might check things like your blood pressure, weight, and give you a general health check.
- They might ask for some tests to make sure everything's good and to catch any issues early on.

After the visit, it's a great idea to keep in touch with your healthcare provider regularly. This way, they can keep an eye on your health, make any tweaks needed and give you the support you need to exercise safely.

2.3 Setting Realistic Goals

Setting goals that are realistic and achievable can make a big difference in having a healthy and happy pregnancy journey. Here's how you can go about it:

Be Specific: Figure out what you want to achieve. For instance, if it's about exercising, be clear on what type of exercise you want to do and how often.

Start Small: Don't rush! It's okay to start with baby steps. Begin with manageable goals that you can comfortably work on without feeling overwhelmed. Gradually increase them as you go along.

Be Flexible: Understand that your body is changing, especially during pregnancy. Be open to adjusting your goals based on how you're feeling. It's okay to modify your plans if needed.

Stay Positive: Focus on the positives! Celebrate your achievements, no matter how small. Positivity goes a long way in keeping you motivated.

Involve Others: Share your goals with your healthcare provider, partner, or a friend. Having someone to support and encourage you can make it easier to stick to your plans.

Listen to Your Body: Pay attention to what your body tells you. If something doesn't feel right, it's okay to take a break or adjust your goals accordingly.

Health is the Goal: Remember, the ultimate goal is a healthy you and a healthy baby. So, any goals you set should be aimed at promoting your well-being during this special time.

Celebrate Progress: Acknowledge and celebrate your progress! Each step forward is a win and brings you closer to a healthier pregnancy.

Remember, every journey is unique. Setting realistic goals helps you stay on track while adapting to the changes happening during this incredible time. You've got this!

Chapter 3: Exercise Routines for Each Trimester

3.1 First Trimester: Adjustments and Early Exercises

The first three months of pregnancy can be a wild ride of emotions. From elation and pure joy to concern, worry, and even fear as you begin to realize that you're responsible for nourishing, growing, and keeping this tiny soon-to-be human being safe and healthy. As long as you're not considered a high-risk pregnancy, you can continue with your regular exercise routine in the first trimester. The foundation of a well-rounded prenatal fitness routine should include at least 150 minutes of cardiovascular activity each week and 2 to 3 days of strength training exercises that target the major muscle groups.

It should also focus on specific exercises that help make pregnancy easier and prepare you for labor and childbirth. (It may seem far off — but it will be here before you know it!).

One area of importance is to work on body awareness to prepare for changes in your posture. Doing an exercise like the pelvic curl is a great way to begin working on spinal mobility and strengthening the abdominal muscles that will support your belly as it grows.

Pelvic Curl

- Lie on your back with your knees bent and feet flat on the ground, about hip-width apart.

- Take a deep breath in to prepare, then exhale as you tuck your pelvis (your "hips") so that you're making an impression of your spine on the floor.

- Keep that tucked position as you continue the exhale and roll through the movement so that you are lifting your spine out of that impression, one vertebra at a time.

- Stop when you reach your shoulder blades.

- Inhale at the top of the movement, then exhale as you fold your body back down, placing one vertebra at a time back onto the floor until you get to your starting position on the back of your pelvis (your "hips," as many people will refer to them as).

- Do 12 to 15 reps. For an added challenge, bring your legs all the way together.

Pelvic Brace

Do this throughout pregnancy as long as you don't have pelvic floor symptoms such as painful intercourse or urinary urgency.

- Lie on your back with your knees bent and feet flat on the ground, about hip-width apart.

- Place your pelvis and low back into a "neutral" position. To find this, make sure you're resting on the back of your pelvis and creating a small space in your lower back (your back should not be pressed into the floor).

- Inhale to prepare, then exhale to perform a Kegel contraction by gently closing the openings (the urethra, the vagina, and anus). As you are performing this contraction, notice how your lower abdominal muscles want to work with that.

- Slightly draw the lower abs in with the Kegel. Inhale, relax the abs and pelvic floor, exhale and repeat contraction.

- Do 2 sets of 8 to 15 repetitions of 3- to 5-second holds, once or twice a day.

Kneeling Push Ups

This move targets core and upper body strengthening together.

- Lie flat on your stomach, then push up onto your hands and knees, keeping your knees behind your hips.

- Pull in your abs (the pelvic brace), and then slowly lower your chest toward the floor as you inhale.

- Exhale as you press back up.

- Start with 6 to 10 and gradually work up to 20 to 24 reps.

Squats

The first trimester is also an ideal time to get squatting! If you have access to the gym, you can also use the leg press machine. Squats, especially bodyweight squats can be done throughout your entire pregnancy. Plus, since squats strengthen all the muscles in your lower body including the quads, glutes, and hamstrings. Keeping these muscles strong is a great way to protect your back, so you use your legs instead of your back when lifting.

- Stand in front of a couch, with your back facing the couch. Begin with feet just wider than hip-width apart. Use the couch as a guide to ensure proper form.

- Squat down like you're about to sit down on the couch, but come back up just as your thighs start to touch it.
- Make sure you take 5 seconds to go down and 3 seconds to come back up.
- Exhale as you squat; inhale as you stand.
- Do 2 sets of 15 to 20 reps.

Bicep Curls

This simple yet effective move is another top pick throughout pregnancy. Bicep curls are a key move to add to your workouts since you need to prep your arms for repeatedly lifting and holding your baby.

- Grab 5- to 10-pound dumbbells and stand with your feet slightly wider than your hips and your knees slightly bent.
- Exhale as you slowly bend your elbows, bringing the dumbbells toward your shoulders.
- Inhale and slowly lower the weights back down.
- Take 3 seconds to lift the dumbbells and 5 seconds to lower.
- Do 2 sets of 10 to 15 repetitions.

Some variations and additional strength training moves to include in the first trimester includes:

- lunges with weight
- glute bridge (if you're experiencing any pelvic pain or have a history of pelvic pain

with pregnancies, you can also add ball squeezes in between your thighs during the glute bridges)

- standard push ups

When it comes to what you should avoid during the first trimester, put your high-intensity interval training (HIIT) on hold since it's an easy way to exhaust yourself early in pregnancy. Also, avoid any exercise where you can experience trauma, such as contact sports.

3.2 Second Trimester: Adapting to Changes

Once the reality sets in that you're in this for the long haul, you may notice a feeling of calmness and even an increase in energy over the next several weeks. Many women say this is the trimester where they feel the best, which is why it's an excellent time to focus on your fitness routine. That said, since the uterus is getting bigger, you do need to be a bit more careful with physical activity.

Activities to avoid during the second trimester include any high impact exercise that involves jumping, running, balance, or exhaustion. You also want to avoid any exercise that has you lying on your back for extended periods of time. In addition to the exercises in the first trimester, consider adding some variations to your squat such as narrow squats, single-leg squats, as well as wide stance squats. Incline pushups, which target the chest, triceps, and shoulders, are another move to add during this trimester.

Now that the core foundation has been established, training the core as the abdomen expands is a much easier concept. And with things beginning to shift and grow even more at this time, she often recommends that moms-to-be continue to work on stability and strength with an extra focus on the inner thighs and glutes.

Incline Pushups

- Stand facing a ledge or railing and place your hands shoulder-width apart on the surface.
- Step your body back into a standing plank position with your back in a straight line.
- Bend your arms and slowly lower your chest toward the railing or ledge.
- Straighten your arms to return to the starting position.
- Do 2 sets of 10 to 12 repetitions.

Hip Flexor and Quadriceps Stretch

Due to postural changes, the second trimester is the ideal time to develop a stretching routine that focuses on the hip flexors, quadriceps, low back, gluteals, and calves.

Because of your changing center of gravity, the belly tends to fall forward, creating shortened hip flexor muscles. This exercise allows you to safely stretch during pregnancy.

- Go into a half-kneeling position on the floor. Place your right knee on the floor and your left foot in front of you, left foot flat on the floor.
- Keeping your posture nice and tall, lunge toward your left foot until you feel a stretch in the front of your right hip and thigh.

- Hold for 30 seconds, ease off, and then repeat 2 more times.
- Switch sides and repeat.

Side-Lying Leg Lifts

To prepare for your changing center of gravity, it's important to get the muscles that help with balance and assist in pelvic stabilization stronger.

- Lie on your right side with both knees bent and stacked on top of one another.
- Slightly lift your right side off of the floor to create a small gap between your waist and the floor. This also levels your pelvis.
- Straighten your left leg and angle it slightly in front of you. Rotate your hip so that your toes point down toward the floor.

- Exhale as you take about 3 seconds to lift your leg; inhale for 3 seconds back down. As you lift your leg, make sure you don't lose that little gap you created between your waist and the floor.

- Do 2 sets of 8 to 15 repetitions on each side.

Mermaid Stretch

As your baby grows, it can start to create pressure on your diaphragm and ribs that can be painful.

- Sit on the ground with both of your knees bent (or folded) and your feet facing to the right.

- Raise your left arm straight to the ceiling as you inhale, then exhale and side bend your torso toward the right. The stretch should be felt on the left side in this example. Hold for 4 slow, deep breaths. This would be the direction to stretch if you experience discomfort on the left side.

- Reverse directions for discomfort on the right side. To reduce the risk of this occurring, start stretching both directions during the second trimester.

3.3 Third Trimester: Preparing for Labor and Delivery

You'll definitely notice a slowdown if not an abrupt halt at times during the third trimester, as your body begins to prepare for labor and childbirth. This is a great time to focus on cardiovascular activities and keep up your mobility and abdominal strength with:

- Walking

- Swimming

- Prenatal yoga

- Pilates

- Pelvic floor exercises

- Bodyweight moves

These help to keep your upper and lower body muscles strong.

For safety purposes, avoid any exercise that places you at a risk for falls. Because your center of gravity is changing daily, it's smart to avoid exercises that would lead to a loss of balance, resulting in a fall and possible abdominal impact that could harm your baby. It's also not uncommon to experience pubic symphysis pain, which is pain in the front pubic bone. Because of this, avoid exercises where your legs are too far apart, which will further aggravate this pain.

Diastasis Recti Correction

"Diastasis recti [separation of the rectus abdominal muscles] is a concern for women during this time and it will show up as a bulge that runs down the midline of your abdomen. In order to combat this, engage in a diastasis recti correction exercise.

- Lie on your back with a pillow under your head and shoulders. Knees are bent, and feet are flat on the floor.
- Use a crib or twin sheet and roll it so it's about 3 to 4 inches wide, and place it on your lower back (above your pelvis and below your ribs).
- Grab the sheet and cross it once over your abdomen. Then, grasp the sides, and the sheet should form an X as you pull each side.

- Take a deep breath in to prepare, then press your back flat into the floor as you raise your head and shoulders off of the pillow. During this motion, you are gently "hugging" the sheet around your abdomen to support your abs.
- Inhale lower, and repeat 10 to 20 times. If your neck or shoulders hurt, start at 10 and work your way up.
- Do this 2 times a day.

Other low-weight or bodyweight-only strength training exercises to target during the third trimester include:

- bodyweight squats or sumo squats with a wider stance for an increased base of support (if you're not experiencing pelvic pain)

- standing shoulder press with light weights

- bicep curls with light weights

- pushups against a wall

- modified planks

- tricep kickbacks with light weight

Chapter 4: Cardiovascular Workouts for Pregnancy

4.1 Aerobic Exercise for Stamina and Circulation

Aerobic activity makes you breathe faster and works your heart and muscles harder. It is sometimes called cardiovascular exercise.

Examples of aerobic activities include:

- brisk walking
- dancing
- running
- swimming or aqua aerobics

How Much Aerobic Activity Should I Do?

If you did aerobics before you became pregnant, it is fine to continue for as long as you feel comfortable. Try to do at least 150 minutes of aerobic exercise every week, over 3 or more days.

If you are new to exercise, start more gently and gradually build up to this amount. You may want to start with 10 minutes of low-impact activities, where you keep one foot on the floor throughout the exercise. Examples include knee raises and brisk walking. As you get used to exercising, you can gradually increase your sessions to 30 to 45 minutes of more energetic exercises.

4.2 Low-Impact Cardio Options

Your body doesn't have to take a beating to get a great cardio workout. Instead, you can always try doing low-impact cardio workouts that are easier on the body. But that doesn't mean that low-impact cardio workouts are more accessible than rounds of burpees or box jumps.

Low-Impact Cardio Exercises To Try

Not sure if a move is a high or low-impact move? If it's the latter, you'll always have at least one foot on the ground. There are different low-impact exercises a person can do that will get their heart pumping, including:

- walking
- muscle-strengthening exercises (e.g., some yoga poses)
- tai chi, an activity that features slow movements and controlled breathing

But you can also consider doing some of the following moves. Feel free to do each exercise in order and repeat the whole set one to two more times. And for a challenge, increase the resistance (via dumbbells, resistance bands, etc.) while doing the moves if it is safe for you to do so based on healthcare provider guidance.

Lateral Lunge to Reach
Strengthens glutes, abductor muscles, adductor muscles and hamstrings.

To do this exercise:

- Stand with feet close together and hands by sides.
- Keeping the chest lifted, take a big step to the side with your left leg.
- Send your butt back, keeping the right leg straight, and bend your left knee to form a 90-degree angle. Your feet should be facing forward.
- Reach your right arm to touch the left foot and raise your left arm straight overhead.

- Push off left foot to return to starting position.
- Repeat for 22 seconds, then switch sides.

Sumo Squat Touch-Down to Heel Raise
Strengthens the glutes, abductor muscles, adductor muscles, hamstrings and calves.

To do this exercise:

- Start standing with feet a little wider than shoulder distance apart and toes turned out slightly.
- Straighten your arms in front of your hips.
- Keeping chest lifted, core braced, and back straight, bend both knees, send butt back and down, and touch hands to the floor.

- Press feet into the ground to stand back up, lifting heels off the ground and arms overhead with legs straight.
- Repeat for 45 seconds.

Plank Walk-out to Push-up
Strengthens the shoulders, arms, core, back, and chest.

To do this exercise:

- Start standing with feet hip-distance apart and hands by your sides.
- Fold your torso forward to bring hands to the ground, slightly bending the knees.
- Walk hands forward into a high plank, with shoulders over wrists.
- Keeping shoulders back and down and tucking pelvis to brace the core, lower

chest toward the ground to do a push-up, bending elbows at 45 degrees.

- Press your hands into the ground to push back up into a high plank.
- Walk hands back toward feet and roll up to standing.
- Repeat for 45 seconds.

Repeater

Strengthens the hamstrings, quads, and glutes

To do this exercise:

- Stand with your right foot forward with a slight bend in the knee and your left foot back on a slight diagonal from your right foot on the ground.
- Lean torso slightly to the right, hinging forward with a straight spine and braced core to align over the right leg.

- Raise arms overhead.

- Simultaneously drive the left knee up and bring hands down to touch (parallel to waist), squeezing abs.

- Bring your left foot back to the ground behind you, straightening your leg, and raising your arms overhead.

- Repeat for about 22 seconds, then switch sides.

Front Kick to Touch Back

Strengthens the hamstrings and glutes

To do this exercise:

- Start standing with feet hip-width apart and hold fists by cheekbones in a guard position.

- Kick your right leg forward straight out in front of you.

- Place your right foot back down and step left foot back in a low lunge while your left-hand touches the ground in front of you and the right-hand rest on the back.

- Repeat for about 22 seconds, then switch sides.

Elevator Plank

Strengthens the shoulders, arms, core and back

To do this exercise:

- Start in a high plank with shoulders stacked over wrists and legs extended behind you.

- Tuck pelvis in to brace core and squeeze glutes and quads.

- Keeping hips lifted and steady, lower right elbow to the ground, followed by your left elbow to get into a forearm plank.
- Place your right hand on the ground to straighten your elbow, followed by your left hand to get back into a high plank.
- Keep your core tight to avoid dipping the hips to one side as you lower down into a forearm plank and come back up into a high plank.
- Repeat for 45 seconds.

Russian Twist With Punch

Strengthens the abs, obliques, arms, and shoulders

To do this exercise:

- Sit on the ground with knees bent and feet flat.

- Lean your torso back about 45 degrees or until you feel abs engaged, then lift your feet off the ground.
- Without moving your legs, rotate the torso to the right, then punch your left arm to the right.
- Return to center and rotate torso to the left, then punch right arm to the left.
- Continue alternating for 45 seconds.

Skier

Strengthens the hamstrings, calves, quads, shoulders, and lats.

To do this exercise:

- Stand with feet together and come up to balls of feet with heels off the ground and arms overhead.

- Squeeze fists to create tension in the arms and shoulders.
- Push hips back, bend knees, and hinging your torso forward until it's almost parallel to the ground, keeping the spine straight and bringing heels to the ground.
- At the same time, swing your arms down and behind you.
- Then, thrust your hips forward and swing your arms overhead, coming back to your toes.
- Repeat for 45 seconds.

4.3 Guidelines for Safe Cardiovascular Workouts

Frequency: 5 times per week

Intensity: Warm up for 5 minutes. Then do moderate-intensity activity, making sure you can pass the "talk test" - that is, the exercise is not so intense that you cannot converse with someone else. Cool down for 5 minutes.

Time: Exercise for at least 10 minutes at a time, with a goal of at least 30 minutes per day (more is even better, if tolerated).

Type: any activity that raises your heart rate for at least 10 minutes, such as walking, bicycling, jogging, swimming, vacuuming, scrubbing, shoveling, etc.

Don't forget to add strength training and stretching to your exercise program as well. Remember: you should discuss your exercise plan and fitness goals with your physician before you begin.

Chapter 5: Strength Training and Flexibility Exercises

5.1 Safe Resistance Training During Pregnancy

Lifting weights is one of the best ways to minimize pregnancy aches and pains. It's also an excellent way to stay fit, build strength for labor, and help prepare you for the physical demands that come with having a baby. If you're already well-versed in strength training, you may already have a set routine that you can stick to during pregnancy with some modifications as your body changes, of course.

Can You Lift Weights While Pregnant?

The short answer is yes, you can lift weights while pregnant. In fact, the American College of

Obstetricians and Gynecologists (ACOG) recommends aerobic and strength conditioning exercises for most people with uncomplicated pregnancies. Research suggests that even heavy resistance training including Olympic level weightlifting does not negatively impact pregnancy outcomes or pelvic floor health. Still, most experts advise certain precautions when weight training while pregnant. For one, you should avoid lying on your back for long periods. You should also forgo overhead lifting since this motion can increase your spine curve and cause lower back pain. If you're newer to strength training, consider using weight machines over free weights. Weight machines are ideal, especially for gym newbies, because they control your range of motion and can provide support. Alternatively, resistance bands are an affordable and portable choice. If you're accustomed to doing free-weight exercises, you may be able to continue during pregnancy with some modifications. Talk to a health care provider to be sure your routine is safe for your abdominal muscles and changing body.

Researchers have found that strengthening exercises can also improve energy levels and reduce fatigue. Resistance training during pregnancy supplements aerobic activity and strengthens muscles in a way cardiovascular exercise does not.

Here are the benefits of weight training when you're expecting.
Strengthens Back Muscles: Lower back pain is a common complaint during pregnancy, affecting approximately two-thirds of all pregnant people. This is because a growing uterus and enlarged

breasts can shift your center of gravity and increase the curvature of your back, which puts extra strain on the back muscles. Lifting weights can strengthen back muscles and increase core strength, which helps support the additional weight of your changing body.

Easier Labor: Research shows that exercise, particularly resistance training, has a positive effect on labor outcomes. It can decrease the chance of cesarean delivery and decrease the length of a hospital stay, lower the chance of an instrumental delivery and shorten the early stages of labor.

And try not to worry about going into early labor because of your workout, studies also show that resistance exercises do not increase the risk of preterm labor.

Better Weight Management: Pregnancy weight gain is expected and important to support the growth of your baby. Too much weight gain, however, may lead to health problems, like gestational diabetes and hypertension while increasing the risk of obesity in your child. It can also increase your risk of obesity after pregnancy. Too little weight gain can lead to your child being too small, this increases their risk of illness and may lead to developmental delays.

5.2 Core Strengthening and Pelvic Floor Exercises

You can activate the pelvic floor anytime, anywhere. But it's also beneficial to incorporate specific exercises that strengthen and target the pelvic floor muscles. One way to design a program is to categorize the exercises for those who have hypotonic pelvic floor muscles versus those who have hypertonic pelvic floor muscles.

Hypotonic means you have low tone pelvic floor issues and need to strengthen and improve endurance and power. Hypertonic means your pelvic floor muscles are too tight or overactive and need to lengthen and relax the muscles.

Exercises for Hypotonic Pelvic Floor Muscles
To target hypotonic pelvic floor issues, three exercises are recommended.

Quick flick Kegels: The quick flick Kegel requires quick contractions of your pelvic floor to help activate the muscles faster and stronger to stop leaks upon sneezing or coughing.

- Begin by lying on the floor with your knees bent and feet flat on the floor. As this exercise becomes easier, try sitting or standing while performing it.
- Find your pelvic floor muscles using the tips described above.
- Exhale, pull your navel to your spine, and quickly contract and release your pelvic floor muscles. Aim to contract for 1 second before releasing.
- Maintain steady breathing throughout.
- Repeat the quick flick 10 times, then rest for 10 seconds. Do 2–3 sets.

Heel Slides: Heel slides encourage pelvic floor contractions while targeting the deep abdominal muscles.

- Begin by lying on the floor with your knees bent and pelvis in a neutral position.

- Inhale into the rib cage, then exhale through the mouth, letting your ribs naturally compress.

- Draw your pelvic floor up, lock in your core, and slide your right heel away from you. Only go as far as you can without losing your connection to your deep core.

- Find the bottom position, then inhale and bring your leg back to the starting position.

- Repeat.

- Do 10 slides up and back and then repeat with the other leg.

Marches (Toe Taps): Like heel slides, the marching exercise increases core stability and encourages pelvic floor contractions.

- Begin by lying on the floor with your knees bent and pelvis in a neutral position.
- Inhale into your rib cage, then exhale through your mouth, letting your ribs naturally compress.
- Draw your pelvic floor up and lock in your core.
- Slowly lift one leg up to a tabletop position.
- Slowly lower this leg to the starting position.
- Repeat the movement, alternating legs. You should not feel any pain in your lower back. It's important that your deep core

stays engaged throughout the entire exercise.

- Alternate legs for 12–20 times total.

Exercises for Hypertonic Pelvic Floor Muscles
Hypertonic exercises may provide some relaxation and lengthening for someone who has short or tight pelvic floor muscles. The goal is to lengthen and relax the hypertonic muscles, so contractions are more effective and the muscles can work effectively.

Here are two recommended hypertonic exercises Happy Baby Pose: The Happy Baby Pose is a great addition to a pelvic floor routine when stretching and releasing are the goal.

- Begin by lying on the floor with your knees bent.

- Bring your knees toward your belly at a 90-degree angle, with the soles of your feet facing up.

- Grab and hold the outside or inside of your feet.

- Open your knees until they're slightly wider than your torso. Then, bring your feet up toward your armpits. Make sure your ankles are over your knees.

- Flex your heels and push your feet into your hands. You can stay in this position for several breaths or gently rock from side to side.

Diaphragmatic Breathing: Diaphragmatic breathing encourages the functional relationship between the diaphragm and pelvic floor. It may also help reduce stress.

- Begin by lying flat on the floor on a yoga or exercise mat. You can also perform the exercise in a seated position.

- Do a few seconds of progressive relaxation. Focus on releasing the tension in your body.

- Once relaxed, put one hand on your stomach and the other on your chest.

- Inhale through your nose to expand your stomach, your chest should stay relatively still. Then, breathe in for 2–3 seconds and exhale slowly.

- Repeat several times while keeping one hand on the chest and one on the stomach.

5.3 Stretching and Flexibility Workouts

Stretching is something you probably know you should be doing. It's also the part of the workout that's very easy to skip. You may think you don't have time for it or don't need it. But a stretch session is one of the best ways to end any workout.

Some stretching and flexibility workouts you should consider:

Quad Stretch:

- Stand and hold onto a wall or the back of a chair for balance if needed.
- Grab the top of the left foot and bend your knee, bringing the foot towards the glutes, knee pointing straight at the floor. You should feel a stretch down the front of your leg.
- Squeeze your hips forward for a deeper stretch.
- Hold for 15 to 30 seconds and switch sides, repeating one to three times per leg.

Standing Hamstring Stretch :

- Take your left foot forward and tip from the hips, keeping the back flat.
- Lower down until you feel a stretch in the back of the leg.
- Rest the hands on the upper thighs to give your back some support.
- Hold for 15 to 30 seconds and switch sides, repeating one to three times.

If you feel shaky or your hamstrings are tight, try using a resistance band to give you more leverage.

Chest and Shoulder Stretch:

- Sit or stand and clasp your hands together behind your back, arms straight.

- Lift your hands towards the ceiling, going only as high as is comfortable. You should feel a stretch in your shoulders and chest.
- Hold for 15 to 30 seconds, repeating one to three times.

If your shoulders are a little tight, try just taking your arms behind you and out to the sides like an airplane.

Upper Back Stretch:
- Clasp your hands together in front of you and round your back, pressing your arms away from your body to feel a stretch in your upper back.
- Contract the abs to get the most out of this stretch.
- Hold for 15 to 30 seconds, repeating one to three times.

Biceps Stretch:

- Take your arms out to the sides, slightly behind you, with your thumbs up, like a hitchhiker.
- Rotate your thumbs down and back until they are pointing to the back wall to stretch the biceps.
- Hold for 15 to 30 seconds, repeating one to three times.

Shoulder Stretch:

- Take your right arm straight across your chest and curl the left hand around your elbow, gently pulling on the right arm to deepen the stretch in the shoulders.
- Try dropping the shoulder down if you're not feeling a stretch.

- Hold for 15 to 30 seconds and switch sides, repeating one to three times on each side.

Seated Side Stretch:

- Sitting or standing, clasp your hands straight up overhead, palms facing the ceiling.
- Stretch up and then over to the right, feeling a stretch down your left side.
- Hold for 15 to 30 seconds and switch sides, repeating one to three times.

Triceps Stretch:

- Bend your right elbow behind your head and use the right hand to gently pull the left elbow in further until you feel a stretch in your triceps.

- Hold for 15 to 30 seconds and switch sides, repeating one to three times.

Chapter 6: Yoga and Mindfulness for Expecting Moms

6.1 Benefits of Prenatal Yoga

Prenatal yoga is a type of yoga designed for pregnant women. Yoga is intended to create a balance between emotional, mental, physical, and spiritual dimensions. Prenatal yoga is about helping you prepare for childbirth by relaxing the body and focusing on safe techniques and poses in all stages of pregnancy.

Yoga can improve your physical and psychological health — and not just for the duration of your pregnancy.

More benefits of doing prenatal yoga include:

Reduces Stress and Symptoms of Depression and Anxiety: The combination of intentional movement and structured breathing can help alleviate symptoms of depression. Breathing in slow, rhythmic breaths activates the nervous system and blocks cortisol, which, in high amounts, has been linked to depresssion.

Improves Blood Flow: The stretching and movements in yoga help increase blood flow to your heart. Improved blood flow means more oxygen-rich blood is going to your baby. This keeps your baby on track for healthy development.

Betters Your Labor Experience: Starting prenatal yoga in any trimester can help you better relax and stay positive once you go into labor. Meditation and breathing exercises have been shown to reduce pain and anxiety during labor. Being confident and building your coping abilities will also help you have a less painful labor experience.

6.2 Relaxation Techniques and Breathing Exercises

Take a deep breath in. Now let it out. You may notice a difference in how you feel already. Your breath is a powerful tool to ease stress and make you feel less anxious. Some simple breathing exercises can make a big difference if you make them part of your regular routine.

Before you get started, keep these tips in mind:

- Choose a place to do your breathing exercise. It could be in your bed, on your living room floor, or in a comfortable chair.

- Don't force it. This can make you feel more stressed.
- Try to do it at the same time once or twice a day.
- Wear comfortable clothes.

Many breathing exercises take only a few minutes. When you have more time, you can do them for 10 minutes or more to get even greater benefits.

Pursed Lip Breathing: This simple breathing technique makes you slow down your breathing pace by having you apply deliberate effort in each breath. You can practice pursed lip breathing at any time. It may be especially useful during activities such as bending, lifting, or stair climbing. Practice using this breath 4 to 5 times a day when you begin so that you can correctly learn the breathing pattern.

To do it:

- Relax your neck and shoulders.

- Keeping your mouth closed, inhale slowly through your nose for 2 counts.

- Pucker or purse your lips as though you were going to whistle.

- Exhale slowly by blowing air through your pursed lips for a count of 4.

Diaphragmatic Breathing: Diaphragmatic breathing (aka belly breathing) can help you use your diaphragm properly. This type of breathing is particularly helpful in people with breathing challenges due to chronic obstructive pulmonary disease (COPD), heart problems, or cancer. It may also help reduce stress and help with challenges related to eating disorders, constipation, high blood pressure, migraine episodes, and other health conditions.

Practice diaphragmatic breathing for 5 to 10 minutes 3 to 4 times daily.

When you begin, you may feel tired, but over time the technique should become easier and should feel more natural.

- Lie on your back with your knees slightly bent and your head on a pillow.
- You may place a pillow under your knees for support.
- Place one hand on your upper chest and one hand below your rib cage, allowing you to feel the movement of your diaphragm.
- Slowly inhale through your nose, feeling your stomach pressing into your hand.

- Keep your other hand as still as possible.

- Exhale using pursed lips as you tighten your abdominal muscles, keeping your upper hand completely still.

You can place a book on your abdomen to make the exercise more difficult. Once you learn how to do belly breathing lying down, you can increase the difficulty by trying it while sitting in a chair. You can then practice the technique while performing your daily activities.

Breath Focus Technique: This deep breathing technique uses imagery or focus words and phrases. You can choose a focus word that makes you smile, feel relaxed, or is simply neutral. Examples include peace, let go, or relax, but it can be any word that suits you to focus on and repeat through your practice. As you build up your breath focus practice, you can start with a 10-minute session. Gradually increase the duration until your sessions are at least 20 minutes.

To do it:

- Sit or lie down in a comfortable place.
- Bring your awareness to your breaths without trying to change how you're breathing.
- Alternate between normal and deep breaths a few times. Notice any differences between normal breathing and deep breathing. Notice how your abdomen expands with deep inhalations.
- Note how shallow breathing feels compared to deep breathing.
- Practice your deep breathing for a few minutes.

- Place one hand below your belly button, keeping your belly relaxed, and notice how it rises with each inhale and falls with each exhale.

- Let out a loud sigh with each exhale.

- Begin the practice of breath focus by combining this deep breathing with imagery and a focus word or phrase that will support relaxation.

- You can imagine that the air you inhale brings waves of peace and calm throughout your body. Mentally say, "Inhaling peace and calm."

- Imagine that the air you exhale washes away tension and anxiety. You can say to yourself, "Exhaling tension and anxiety."

Lion's Breath: Lion's breath is an energizing yoga breathing practice that is said to relieve tension in your chest and face. It's also known in yoga as Lion's Pose.

To do this:

- Come into a comfortable seated position. You can sit back on your heels or cross your legs.
- Press your palms against your knees with your fingers spread wide.
- Inhale deeply through your nose and open your eyes wide.
- At the same time, open your mouth wide and stick out your tongue, bringing the tip down toward your chin.
- Contract the muscles at the front of your throat as you exhale out through your mouth by making a long "haaa" sound.

- You can turn your gaze to look at the space between your eyebrows or the tip of your nose.
- Do this breath 2 to 3 times.

Alternate Nostril Breathing: Alternate nostril breathing is a breathing practice for relaxation. It has been shown to enhance cardiovascular function and lower heart rate. It is best practiced on an empty stomach. Avoid the practice if you're feeling sick or congested. Keep your breath smooth and even throughout the practice.

To do this:
- Choose a comfortable seated position.
- Lift your right hand toward your nose, pressing your first and middle fingers down toward your palm and leaving your other fingers extended.

- After an exhale, use your right thumb to gently close your right nostril.

- Inhale through your left nostril and then close your left nostril with your right pinky and ring fingers.

- Release your thumb and exhale out through your right nostril.

- Inhale through your right nostril and then close this nostril.

- Release your fingers to open your left nostril and exhale through this side.

- This is one cycle.

- Continue this breathing pattern for up to 5 minutes.

- Finish your session with an exhale on the left side.

Equal Breathing: This breathing technique focuses on making your inhales and exhales the same length. Making your breath smooth and steady can help bring about balance and equanimity. You should find a breath length that is not too easy and not too difficult. You also don't want it to be too fast in order to maintain it throughout the practice. Usually, this is between 3 and 5 counts. Once you get used to equal breathing while seated, you can do it during your yoga practice or other daily activities.

To do it:

- Choose a comfortable seated position.
- Breathe in and out through your nose.
- Count during each inhale and exhale to make sure they are even in duration. Alternatively, choose a word or short

phrase to repeat during each inhale and exhale.

- You can add a slight pause for breath retention after each inhale and exhale if you feel comfortable. (Normal breathing involves a natural pause.)
- Continue practicing this breath for at least 5 minutes.

6.3 Mindfulness Practices for Stress Reduction

Mindfulness, the awareness that emerges through paying attention moment by moment without judgement is gaining popularity in many circles for its important role in reducing stress and improving overall health. But just like any habit, mindfulness needs to be practiced regularly to experience its full benefits.

Swimming or Floating in the Water: Swimming uses the entire body without putting pressure on the joints. Bringing movement into stiff and tense areas can release a lot of physical stress. This increases mobility and allows more oxygen to flow into muscles we use less often. Swimming can naturally draw you into a rhythm with your breath as you find your stroke. Immersing yourself in water can eliminate distractions, allowing you to be more mindful of internal states. If swimming isn't manageable, try floating and focus on experiencing the way your body moves in the water as you breathe.

Meditative Walking (Core Walking): The breath, body and mind are all connected. When we can slow down movement and breath, the mind naturally will follow. Moving can make it easier to be present with what we are trying to be mindful of. When we walk, there is a lot of forward momentum involved to drive the body forward. By slowing down and removing the forward drive, we start to use our stabilizing muscles to keep us upright. Strengthening these smaller muscles in the abdomen, or core, can ease body pain in the long run and help with balance.

There are many things to be mindful of during meditative walking, such as keeping your breath relaxed or putting an even amount of weight on each leg. Or perhaps focus on your shoulders moving along without bouncing up and down. This is a good indicator you are taking deeper, fuller breaths from your abdomen, rather than shallow breaths into the chest. Good places to try a walking meditation are a flat area of the beach, hallway or even a few laps around your living room. Just make sure you're eliminating as many distractions for yourself as you can.

Drinking a Cup of Tea: Any activity can become a mindfulness exercise if you take the time to experience it. Take some time to experience the preparation of the tea, the way it smells, the way your arms lift to bring it to your lips and the way the warmth feels in your body. Slowing down the process of drinking a cup of tea or another warm beverage not only can invite you to become more present but also quiets the mental conversation.

Hiking or Connecting with Nature: Being in nature provides an ideal space to disconnect from technology and become more mindful of the senses. Experiencing the crunch of leaves under your feet, the smell of the plants and the sounds of the birds can send signals to your nervous system to relax.

Gazing Meditation: Choose an external object such as a candle flame, the horizon line or a camp fire. Allow your focus to rest softly on your point and settle in. This can be a great way to start practicing mindfulness with your eyes open. (It's OK to blink.) When the urge to look away is resisted, the ability to meditate and be mindful becomes stronger and can provide a very tangible transition into a more balanced, calm state of mind.

Chapter 7: Nutrition and Diet for a Healthy Pregnancy

7.1 Importance of Proper Nutrition During Pregnancy

Generally speaking, there are countless benefits to eating healthy. Just to name a few, a nutritious diet yields a woman more sustainable energy, a stronger immune system, and a reduced risk of disease. Pregnant women need to be particularly careful about what they eat because they are not only eating for their own health, but they are also eating for their baby's health! When a woman eats well during her pregnancy, she reduces the chances of complications such as anemia, low birth weight, and birth defects. Eating well can also help with unpleasant pregnancy symptoms! Below are some other benefits of a healthy pregnancy diet.

Increased Energy: Experiencing a paralyzing amount of fatigue during pregnancy is very common for most women. Sometimes no matter what you do, fatigue is hard to control especially in the early weeks with all the hormonal changes your body is going through. Keeping a wholesome diet and eating every 3-4 hours will keep your energy up. It's important to remember your iron consumption should be doubled when you are pregnant to help sustain your increased blood volume and promote iron storage for the fetus.

Successful Fetal Development: A balanced diet is just what your baby needs to grow correctly. You want to aim at eating at least 300 more calories a day than you normally would. However, you don't want to go overboard as it can lead to complications such as preeclampsia and gestational diabetes. Essential vitamins and nutrients that will warrant a healthy baby include but are not limited to: folate or folic acid, vitamin C, vitamin A, calcium, fiber, fruits and veggies, whole grains, and an adequate amount of protein and fat.

Improved Sleep: Numerous factors can keep you up at night during your pregnancy, such as nausea, late-night bathroom breaks, or aches and pains! Making sure you are eating full and complete meals each day, and staying away from too much caffeine, will definitely help with your beauty rest. The vitamins and minerals that are needed during pregnancy such as vitamin B, calcium, and iron also aid in productive sleep.

Reduced Risk of Getting Sick: Pregnant women are more susceptible to certain infections such as the flu. A healthy diet and plenty of rest can prevent this from happening. Although a minor cold will most likely not affect your baby, suffering from pregnancy symptoms is bad enough and being sick on top of that is not appealing. Trying to avoid getting sick in general is a safe bet!

7.2 Balanced Diet Essentials for Expectant Mothers

While you're pregnant, you'll want to eat extra protein, calcium, iron, and essential vitamins. You can get these by eating a wide variety of lean meat, seafood, whole grains, and plant-based foods.

Here are nutritious foods to eat when you're pregnant to help make sure you're eating healthily.

Dairy products: During pregnancy, you'll need extra protein and calcium to meet your baby's needs. Dairy products like milk, cheese, and yogurt are good choices. Dairy products contain two types of high-quality protein: casein and whey. Dairy is the best dietary source of calcium. It also provides phosphorus, B vitamins, magnesium, and zinc.

Yogurt may also be beneficial. Some varieties also contain probiotic bacteria, which support digestive health.
If you're lactose intolerant, you may also be able to tolerate yogurt, especially probiotic yogurt.

Legumes: These include lentils, peas, beans, chickpeas, soybeans, and peanuts. Legumes are great plant-based sources of fiber, protein, iron, folate, and calcium — all of which your body needs more of during pregnancy.

Folate is one of the most essential B vitamins (B9). It's very important for you and your baby, especially during the first trimester, and even before. You'll need at least 600 micrograms (mcg) of folate every day, which can be a challenge to achieve with foods alone. But legumes can boost your folate levels along with supplementation based on your doctor's recommendation.

Legumes tend to be high in fiber, and some are also high in iron, magnesium, and potassium. Consider adding legumes to your diet with meals like hummus on whole grain toast, black beans in a taco salad, or a lentil curry.

Sweet potatoes: Sweet potatoes are rich in beta-carotene, a plant compound that your body converts to vitamin A. Vitamin A is essential for a baby's development. However, too much vitamin A, from animal products such as organ meats can cause toxicity. Sweet potatoes are a good plant-based source of beta-carotene and fiber. Fiber keeps you full longer, reduces blood sugar spikes, and improves digestive health, which can help reduce the risk of pregnancy constipation. Try sweet potatoes at breakfast time as a base for your morning avocado toast.

Salmon: Smoked on a whole wheat bagel, teriyaki grilled, or served with pesto, salmon is a welcome addition to this list. Salmon is rich in essential omega-3 fatty acids, which have a host of benefits. Omega-3s are present in seafood. They help build the brain and eyes of your baby and may help increase gestational length.

While it's best to avoid some seafoods during pregnancy, due to mercury and other contaminants, salmon, sardines, and anchovies are safe to eat. However, it's worth checking where it was fished from, especially if it was locally caught. It's also best to opt for fresh salmon, as smoked seafood can carry a risk of listeria.

Here are the high mercury fish to avoid:
- Swordfish
- Shark
- King mackerel
- Marlin

* Bigeye tuna

* Tilefish

Eggs: Eggs are a healthy food, as they contain a little of almost every nutrient you need. A large egg contains about 71 calories, 3.6 g of protein, fat, and many vitamins and minerals. Eggs are a great source of choline, a vital nutrient during pregnancy. It's important in a baby's brain development and helps prevent developmental abnormalities of the brain and spine. A single whole egg contains roughly 147 milligrams (mg) of choline, which will get you closer to the current recommended choline intake of 450 mg per day while pregnant, though more studies are underway to determine if that is enough.

Broccoli and Dark, Leafy Greens: Broccoli and dark, green vegetables, such as spinach have many of the nutrients you'll need. If you don't like the flavors, you can disguise them by adding them to soups, pasta sauces, and more.

Benefits include fiber, vitamin C, vitamin K, vitamin A, calcium, iron, folate, and potassium. Their fiber content can also help prevent constipation. Vegetables have also been linked to a reduced risk of low birth weight.

Lean Meat and Proteins: Lean beef, pork, and chicken are excellent sources of high-quality protein. Beef and pork are also rich in iron, choline, and other B vitamins — all of which you'll need in higher amounts during pregnancy. Iron is an essential mineral used by red blood cells as a part of hemoglobin. You'll need more iron since your blood volume is increasing, and especially during your third trimester. Low levels of iron during early and mid-pregnancy may cause iron deficiency anemia, which increases the risk of low birth weight and other complications. It can be hard to cover your iron needs with meals alone, especially if you develop an aversion to meat or follow a plant-based diet. However, for those who can, lean red meat may help increase the amount of iron you're getting from food.

Berries: Berries provide water, healthy carbs, vitamin C, fiber, and antioxidants. They also have a relatively low glycemic index value, so they should not cause significant spikes in blood sugar. Berries are a great snack, as they contain both water and fiber. They provide a lot of flavor and nutrition but with relatively few calories.
Some of the best berries to eat while pregnant are blueberries, raspberries, goji berries,

strawberries, and acai berries. Check out this blueberry smoothie for some inspiration.

Whole Grains: Unlike their refined counterparts, whole grains are packed with fiber, vitamins, and plant compounds. Think oats, quinoa, brown rice, wheat berries, and barley instead of white bread, pasta, and white rice. Some whole grains, like oats and quinoa, also contain a fair amount of protein, as well as B vitamins, fiber, and magnesium.

Avocados: Avocados contain monounsaturated fatty acids. This makes them taste buttery and rich — perfect for adding depth and creaminess to a dish.

They also provide fiber, antioxidants, B vitamins (especially folate), vitamin K, potassium, copper, vitamin E, and vitamin C. Because of their high content of healthy fats, folate, and potassium, avocados are a great choice during pregnancy.

Fish Liver Oil: Fish liver oil is made from the oily liver of fish, usually from cod. It's rich in the omega-3 fatty which is essential for fetal brain and eye development. Supplementing with fish oil may help protect against preterm delivery and may benefit fetal eye development. Fish liver oil is also very high in vitamin D, which many people lack. It may be beneficial if you don't regularly eat seafood or if you don't already supplement with omega-3 or vitamin D.

7.3 Meal Planning and Nutritional Tips

Below is an example of a 7-day meal plan you can follow during pregnancy. The serving sizes may vary depending on your trimester, and a registered dietitian can help you build an eating plan that satisfies your needs.

Day 1

Breakfast - Whole grain toast with cottage cheese, fresh tomato slices, and chives.

Lunch - Mixed bean salad with diced carrot, celery, bell pepper, and avocado. Mix in your favorite tinned fish for protein, and serve whole grain crackers on the side (optional.)

Dinner - BBQ chicken thighs with corn on the cob, grilled onion, and a Mediterranean-inspired quinoa salad (add sundried tomatoes, cubed cucumber, and tomato, and dress with olive oil, lemon juice, fresh garlic, and basil.)

Snacks - Hard-boiled eggs on whole wheat pita; Greek yogurt with fresh fruits and nuts.

Day 2

Breakfast - Baked oatmeal with Greek yogurt, banana, blueberries, whisked eggs, cinnamon, and a drizzle of honey.

Lunch - Chicken noodle soup with a side of green salad. Add fresh herbs to your soup to add additional flavor to your dish.

Dinner - Extra-lean ground beef meatloaf with baked asparagus, broccoli with garlic, and sweet potatoes.

Snacks - Tuna fish and whole grain crackers; cottage cheese with fresh fruits and nuts.

Day 3

Breakfast - A high-fiber cold cereal (minimum 8g per serving) with fresh fruits, a handful of mixed nuts, milk, and a dollop of Greek yogurt.

Lunch - Baked flatbread pizza with whole grain pita bread, feta cheese, roasted chicken breast, tomatoes, onions, and bell peppers.

Dinner - Grilled pork skewers with pineapple and onions. Serve with brown rice, a fresh green salad, and your favorite dressing.

Snacks - Fresh vegetables with dip and a portion of cheese; Greek yogurt with fresh fruits and nuts.

Day 4

Breakfast - Overnight oats with chia seeds, banana slices, crushed peanuts (you can swap in any nut if you don't like peanuts), and a spoonful of dark chocolate nibs.

Lunch - Chickpea curried stew with canned tomatoes, potato, carrots, cauliflower, onion, and garlic. Serve with whole-grain naan.

Dinner - Baked salmon crusted with panko crumbs and honey mustard. Serve with boiled potatoes and a fresh salad with your favorite greens and dressing.

Snacks - Avocado dip with whole grain crackers, fresh apple with nut butter.

Day 5

Breakfast - Savory egg omelet with cooked bell peppers, black beans, and avocado mash. Season with your favorite herbs and serve with whole-grain toast.

Lunch - Vegetarian sandwich with whole grain bread. Add lettuce, cucumber slices, red onion, tomato, and hummus. Serve with fresh fruit on the side.

Dinner - Baked sesame crispy tofu served over brown rice. Add sweet onion, cooked eggplant, zucchini, shredded cabbage, and garnish with sesame seeds.

Snacks - Homemade blueberry muffins made with whole wheat flour, walnuts, and ground flax seed; fresh cut vegetables and hummus.

Day 6

Breakfast - Whole grain English muffins with egg, avocado, slices of cheese, and baby arugula for greens. Add mustard for extra flavor.

Lunch - Large shredded salad with kale, Brussels sprouts, sweet onion, blueberries, almonds, feta cheese, almonds, and roasted chicken. Dress with your favorite salad dressing.

Dinner - Stir fry with cabbage, red peppers, onion, fresh mango slices, peanuts, and cilantro. Add cooked shrimp for protein and fresh chili as tolerated. Serve over brown rice.

Snacks - Greek yogurt with fresh fruits and nuts; whole-grain crackers with tinned salmon and cucumber slices.

Day 7

Breakfast - Oatmeal with mixed nuts, berries, a dash of cinnamon, and a dollop of Greek yogurt.

Lunch - Egg salad pita wraps with spinach and sundried tomato. Serve with a small vegetable soup on the side.

Dinner - Whole grain penne pasta with red sauce, ground turkey, and bell peppers. Serve with a green salad on the side.

Snacks - Cottage cheese with fruits and nuts; vegetable sticks with hummus.

Chapter 8: Managing Common Pregnancy Discomforts

8. 1 Dealing with Back Pain and Postural Changes

Throughout pregnancy, hormones affect a woman's muscles and joints. The hormones relaxin and progesterone relax muscles and loosen ligaments and joints, especially in the pelvic area. The extra weight and body changes in pregnancy along with these loosened joints and ligaments can cause discomfort and even lead to injury.

As your uterus grows and becomes heavier, your center of gravity changes. This can lead to problems with balance and the potential for falls. The weight of your baby and weakening of belly muscles pulls your lower spine forward, adding strain to back muscles. Many women respond by leaning back in an awkward posture. This increases back strain and pain.

To prevent back pain:

- Try using proper body mechanics. For example, if you need to pick something up, squat down, bend at your knees and keep your back straight. Avoid bending over from your waist.

- Use good posture when sitting or standing and do back-strengthening exercises. Ask your healthcare provider about back exercises that are right for you.

- Avoid activities that strain the back, like lifting and moving heavy objects.

- Wear shoes that provide good support.

- Sleep on your side with pillows between your knees for support.

- Apply heat, cold, or massage to the painful area.

- If you are having discomfort, talk with your healthcare provider. Back pain relief may need rest, supportive garments, or other types of treatment.

Prevention and treatment of back pain are important to avoid injury and to decrease the chance for long-term or chronic back pain because back pain in pregnancy can be a symptom of more serious problems like preterm labor.

8.2 Exercises to Relieve Discomforts

Here are two minutes exercises to perform to relieve discomforts

- Breathe deeply through your belly; 30 to 60 seconds.

- Stretch hamstrings; 30 seconds.

- Stretch calves; 30 seconds.

- Squeeze a ball between knees; 5-second squeezes, for 60 total seconds.

- Perform seated straight leg raises; 30 seconds each leg.

- March in place; 30 to 60 seconds.

- Walk forward and backward; 10 steps each way.

- Circle arms backward; 30 seconds.

- Moving your arms on a tabletop as if you're doing the breaststroke; 60 seconds.

- Perform wrist circles, wrist bends (up and down), and open and close fingers; 10 seconds each.

8.3 Tips for Better Sleep and Relaxation

Keep Noise Levels Low: Keep your sleep environment as quiet as possible. Also try experimenting with earplugs while you sleep. You might be waking up from noise more often than you think.

Use Light to Your Advantage: Avoiding blue light and bright lights before bed helps regulate your circadian rhythm and prepares you for sleep. Dim your bedroom lights before bedtime to help.

Pick the Right Mattress: Even with the proper schedule, you won't sleep well if you aren't comfortable. See if your mattress is too old, too small, or doesn't support your body where needed. You can also consider adding a mattress topper for more comfort.

Ditch Electronics an Hour Before Bed: By opting for more meditative and relaxing activities before bed, you avoid being overstimulated by electronics. Otherwise, you may have a harder time falling asleep and may have more restless sleep.

Use the Bedtime Relaxation Method: Whether it's soundscapes, a sleep story podcast, or a guided meditation, there is something relaxing for everyone. So use a right bedtime that works for you.

Avoid the Bedroom Until Bedtime: Sleep is more challenging if you've been sitting on your bed studying or watching TV all day. Avoid the bedroom (or at least your bed) until about 1 hour before bed.

Try Aromatherapy: Aromatherapy — surrounding yourself with pleasant or calming smells — can help the body relax by easing anxiety and stress. Speak with a healthcare provider to find a type of aromatherapy that is safe and effective for you.

Hydrate Long Before Sleeping: Drinking water late at night will cause you to make multiple trips to the bathroom. Take only small sips 1 to 2 hours prior to sleeping.

Avoid Alcohol 4 Hours Before Bed: Experts recommend avoiding alcohol at least 4 hours before bedtime. Although alcohol may make you

feel relaxed, it's linked to poor sleep duration
and quality.

Chapter 9: Partner Involvement and Support

9.1 Engaging Partners in Prenatal Fitness

When it comes to prenatal fitness, involving your partner can add a whole new dimension to your journey. Here's how teaming up with your significant other can enrich this special phase:

Team Spirit: Consider making workouts a joint effort. Being each other's cheerleader during exercises fosters support and encouragement. Sharing this experience strengthens the bond and makes fitness a shared accomplishment.

Shared Moments: Exploring fitness activities together creates lasting memories. Whether it's a brisk walk in nature, practicing yoga, or even preparing healthy meals as a team, these shared moments foster a sense of togetherness.

Healthier Habits: Incorporating fitness into your routine often leads to embracing healthier lifestyle habits. It's more than just exercising; it's about making better choices in meals, sleep routines, and stress management, collectively benefiting both of you.

Emotional Support: Your partner's involvement provides crucial emotional support during this journey. Having someone to share both the challenges and victories helps navigate the ups and downs of pregnancy more smoothly.

Engaging Together: Consider participating in workouts, planning nutritious meals, and exploring relaxation techniques as a couple.

These joint activities not only promote fitness but also deepen your connection.

Communication and Togetherness: Open communication lays the foundation for a shared fitness journey. Understanding each other's needs and preferences helps tailor activities that suit both partners, fostering unity and togetherness.

Bonding Beyond Fitness: Apart from workouts, engaging in activities you both enjoy strengthens your relationship. Attending classes, sharing experiences, or simply spending quality time together nurtures your bond.

9.2 Emotional Support and Encouragement

Many expectant and new mothers have a strong sense of responsibility during and after their pregnancies and they put in all the effort to manage all the tasks, like taking care of themselves, the baby, and their home. As a result, they may feel anxious and overwhelmed. However, partner's and family's support can help her experience a smooth pregnancy. You can do things like:

- Help her make changes to her lifestyle
- Show affection
- Take walks together
- Lend a helping hand when she needs
- Encourage her to eat healthy
- Encourage her to take breaks and naps

Women are more likely to enjoy this beautiful time when they have the support they require. They will also be better prepared to deal with the difficulties of being a new mother and develop a positive relationship with their baby.

Why Is Emotional Support and Encouragement Necessary?

- Pregnant women who receive emotional support experience fewer pregnancy difficulties and deliver healthier newborns.
- Lack of emotional support and encouragement during pregnancy increases the risk of stress, anxiety, and depression, all of which can affect the mother's and the child's health.
- Pregnant women feel happier and more at ease by getting emotional support from family, friends, or a therapist, which benefits the unborn child.

- Regular emotional support increases the pregnant woman's likelihood of breastfeeding, which is healthy for both mother and child.

How Can a Partner Be Supportive?

Usually, men want to help their pregnant partners but are unsure how to get involved and what their partner wants or needs. Here are some things you, as a supportive partner can do.

Educate Yourself: Start educating yourself about pregnancy. The more you understand what all changes your partner's body is undergoing and how it is affecting her mental and physical states, you'll be able to provide the right kind of support at the right time. The same is true to get ready for childbirth and postpartum.

Here Are a Few Things You Can Do:

- Get hold of some good pregnancy books. The paperbacks will give detailed information on pregnancy and the stages an expecting and new mother goes through.

- Attend a childbirth class or make an appointment with a childbirth educator or your partner's healthcare provider.

- If you have a friend who has recently delivered a baby, speak with them and understand their journey. Inquire about what they did in a specific situation(s).

Be With Her at All Important Times:

- Attend all of your partner's medical appointments.

- Participate in decisions about which is the best healthcare provider and which prenatal and postnatal tests to undergo.
- Attend childbirth or parenting classes

Talk to Her: When it comes to partner support, open communication is the key. Pregnancy can induce a wide range of emotions from excitement and happiness to fear and anxiety. You will be able to provide the emotional support your partner requires if they can trust that you will listen to their feelings with an open mind and that nothing is off-limits.

Ask the Right Questions: You can't always be aware of what your partner requires. So, do not hesitate before asking your partner what you can do for her. There are many ways to help them and make them feel loved from making sure they have doctor appointments scheduled to giving them back rubs to preparing their favorite nutritious food. However, do not put the burden on your partner and expect them to tell you exactly what to do at every step of the way. Taking proactive actions to support your partner is a crucial component of a supportive relationship.

9.3 Bonding Activities for Couples

Having a baby is an exciting, meaningful, and inevitably life-changing experience for couples. That bun won't be in the oven forever, so take advantage of the alone time you've got left with a date night. Looking for some fun activities for pregnant couples? From massages to movie nights, staycations to mocktails. We rounded up fun date ideas that can help kindle romance and strengthen any relationship.

Take a Hike: A slow-paced walk in nature can improve circulation and ease stress. Make it more romantic by choosing a route with great lookout points—they're perfect for taking breaks (and stealing a kiss).

Try Golfing: Whether it's hitting the driving range or playing a round of mini-golf, both partners will be sure to get a kick out of how the baby bump affects your swing.

Have a Media-Free Moment: Quiet conversations are hard to come by, and that will only become more true after the baby comes. For now, try hiding the smart phones and tablets, turn off the TV, and just talk. You can make it as deep or lighthearted as you want. Try talking about your day, your favorite childhood memories, or even something you're looking forward to teaching your baby.

Book a Couple's Massage: Pregnancy can be stressful—from tying up loose ends at work to feeling anxious about giving birth, and even just carrying around all that extra weight. And chances are your partner is feeling it, too. Make an appointment for some much-needed relaxation and lean into the pre-baby bliss.

Go Out for Dessert: Fancy dinners are great, but nothing says indulgence like a decadent dessert. Have your main meal at home, then get dressed up and head to a fancy spot for something sweet. It will still feel like a big night out, but the bill won't eat into your future diaper budget.

Buy Dinner Ingredients at a Farmer's Market: Pick up some fresh and seasonal produce at your local farmers' market before heading home to whip up something delicious for dinner. If it's warm out, take your delectable creation outside and dine in the backyard.

Catch a Live Show: You don't have to go far to enjoy live theater. Check out a dramatic production at your community theater or laugh yourself silly at a local comedy club. You'll be amazed at how talented your neighbors are!

Go to the Movies: Dinner and a movie is just about the most classic date idea in history, but having a baby will definitely make it more complicated. Head out to see the latest flick with a bucket of popcorn and a bag of M&M's for some good old-fashioned fun.

Plan a Staycation: Travel is certainly possible when pregnant, but comes with its own complications. Indulge in a night or weekend-long stay at a fancy hotel without having to go far for the ultimate (local) babymoon. Try out the spa, check out a bucket list restaurant, or just spend the whole time in bed.

Listen to Live Music: Loud noises and babies don't really mix, so take advantage of being baby-free for a little while longer with a concert. Choose an event that suits your personal taste, whether it's your favorite singer at a sold-out arena or a soothing jazz band at a local venue.

Enroll in a Class: It's never too late to learn something new, and one of the best ways to do that is by taking a class. From dance classes to art, cooking, and more, there are endless things to learn together.

Host a Game Night: Simply hanging at home can be a great way to spend quality time with your partner, and playing board games will enrich the experience. Challenge your partner to a competitive game of Scrabble, or show off your flirty side with a round of "Never Have I Ever."

Chapter 10: Postpartum Fitness and Recovery

10.1 Transitioning to Postpartum Exercise

No matter how fit you were before and even during pregnancy, postpartum exercise presents a unique set of challenges. Your body is still healing from delivery, and with a newborn in the house, you might be feeling more tired than ever. But finding time to fit in fitness is amazing for both your body and mind—it can be just what you need to get back to feeling like your pre-pregnancy self. No, we're not talking about "getting your body back." We're talking about a boost to your energy, self-confidence and physical strength. Plus, you're bound to sleep better too.

Postnatal exercise brings a host of positive benefits to your body, but also for your mood and stress levels. Fitness not only helps your body heal but also provides an outlet to recenter and focus on yourself—something that might feel a bit out of reach now that you're caring for another tiny human. Consistent exercise post-baby provides a huge boost in not only physical strength, but mental strength as well. You just went through so many changes, things have shifted. Exercise helps you heal from the inside out.

In addition to the many mental and emotional benefits, postnatal fitness can lead to weight loss, improved strength (carrying around a baby all the time is no joke), better sleep and more balanced hormones, a must after nine months of ups and downs.

First things first, don't jump into a postpartum exercise routine without your doctor's approval. Many doctors recommend waiting six to eight weeks after birth before starting trying any type of exercise, but it often varies. Some women may experience complications during pregnancy or labor that might set them back a few more weeks. For example, a mother who had a vaginal birth will likely have a different timeline than one who had a c-section. And others may even be able to work out sooner than six weeks. No matter what, it's crucial to work with your doctor to find out exactly when it is right for you and your body. A doctor will be able to check for an indication of diastasis recti (the separation of the abdominals) and be able to recommend the appropriate physical work to heal that or any other side effects of childbirth.

There's no real reason to rush back into exercising early anyways. In fact, it can cause you more harm than good down the line. It might be hard for women used to high intensity workouts or long runs, but taking it slow is key.

When you're ready, start by adding walking and low-impact bodyweight exercises at first. It covers core, strength training, outdoor walking and elliptical, and places special emphasis on healing the pelvic floor muscles and not aggravating a diastasis recti, both of which are crucial for new moms with recovering bodies. Don't worry, you'll gradually work your way back to sprints and burpees in no time.

10.2 Recovery Exercises and Timeliness

You can start this exercise routine the first day after your baby is born. Start with doing each exercise two times a day. Each day do one more repetition per set until you are doing 10 of each exercise two times a day.

Deep Breathing with Abdominal Wall Tightening:

Position: Lying on your back or side with knees bent.

- Take a deep breath through your nose. Let your abdominal wall expand upward.
- With your lips slightly parted, blow air out through your mouth while tightening your abdominal wall.
- Keep blowing until you have emptied your lungs.

- Don't take too many deep breaths in a row or you might get dizzy.

Toe Pointing:

Position: Sitting or lying.

- Pull your toes toward you as far as you can.

- Point your foot downward.

- Repeat.

- Rest before continuing. If pointing your toes downward causes cramps: pull up your toes and relax.

Foot and Ankle Circles:

Position: Sitting or lying.

- Make large, slow circles with each foot, first to the right, then to the left. This is an excellent exercise to improve the circulation in your legs.

Pelvic Tilt

Position: Lying flat on your back with your knees bent and your fleet flat on the bed or floor.

- Tilt your pelvis back by flattening your lower back against the bed or floor.
- Tighten your abdominal muscles and your bottom.

This exercise strengthens your abdominal muscles and helps relieve backache.

10.3 Adjusting to New Fitness Routines

It can feel overwhelming to experience body changes, to not be able to do the things we used to do, especially if we're also coping with body image issues, toxic messaging from diet culture, and mental health struggles. For example, if we're navigating postpartum anxiety or feeling out of control in other areas of our life, we might try to become rigid or strict about exercise or eating. It almost feels comforting to try to anchor ourselves in something consistent when we feel like we're free-falling. But we can easily slip into an unhealthy mindset when this happens.

It's important to stay flexible, listen to our bodies, and adjust our goals when necessary. We have new limitations and challenges after we enter motherhood—physical, mental, and even time limitations. Letting go of perfectionism or all-or-nothing thinking can be helpful.

We don't have to feel like we aren't doing enough, we can embrace what we can accomplish. Adjusting our standards and changing our mindset about exercise can be a good thing.

If you're reading this book on fit mom, healthy baby, you may also be interested in my book on heart disease and lung cancer. Tap the links above to read them.

Thank you for purchasing my book. I'll really appreciate if you could take a moment to leave a review. Your feedback will help me improve and make my next book even better. I'm always looking forward to improving, so please do not hold back! Thank you for your time and support.